How To Do A Handstand

From The Basic Exercises To The Free Standing Handstand Pushup

Patrick Barrett

CONTENTS

"Did you ever notice when you see a group of strong men together that, sooner or later, they take time out for some handbalancing?"

-York Handbalancing Course No. 1, circa 1950

Other Books by Patrick Barrett:

Natural Exercise: Basic Bodyweight Training and Calisthenics for Strength and Weight-Loss

The Natural Diet: Simple Nutritional Advice For Optimal Health In The Modern World

One Arm Pull Up: Bodyweight Training And Exercise Program For One Arm Pull Ups And Chin Ups

INTRODUCTION TO HANDSTAND TRAINING

My name is Patrick Barrett, and I would like to thank you for buying this book. I hope you are able to use it to master the various handstand techniques covered inside, and to improve your strength and balance significantly along the way.

I'm really glad that you decided to learn how to do handstands. Decades ago, handstands and handbalancing were a standard part of training for almost anyone who lifted weights or was interested in getting stronger and healthier.

However, things have changed drastically. Many people prefer the ultra-controlled exercises made possible by machines, and they stay away from exercises like the handstand that require a little more effort to master.

It seems that more "old-school" exercises like the handstand may be starting to make a comeback, and I'm glad you've decided to be a part of that.

I especially like training for exercises like the handstand because not only are you getting stronger, you're also developing a new skill. That makes the training much more interesting and enjoyable, and it's much less mind-numbing than a lot of other hyper-repetitive, mindless workouts that many people do.

Bear in mind that it can also mean you'll get a little bit frustrated in the beginning. If you want to exercise on a machine, all you need to do is find out how it works and you can pretty much sit right down and start using it. You're an 'expert' by the time you do your third rep.

Handstands, and exercises that train you for the handstand, aren't like that—they require a bit more effort and persistence. You're going to learn several exercises in this book, and each one takes time to learn and master.

Mastering those exercises will go much more quickly if you practice them intelligently. We'll discuss that more as we get to the exercises themselves, but keep it in mind—this is not a mindless, repetitive exercise. Pay attention, think about what you're doing, and you'll make better progress.

Let's get started.

Books by Patrick Barrett:

Natural Exercise: Basic Bodyweight Training and Calisthenics for Strength and Weight-Loss

The Natural Diet: Simple Nutritional Advice For Optimal Health In The Modern World

One Arm Pull Up: Bodyweight Training And Exercise Program For One Arm Pull Ups And Chin Ups

BREATHING

Breathing is an important part of handstand training, as it is an important part of any training. Almost any martial artist or athlete will tell you that your breath is your power, and that is as true here as in any other type of physical training.

As a general rule, you will exhale during the more difficult part of an exercise, and inhale during the less difficult part. Put more simply, exhale during exertion.

There are exceptions to any rule, but that's still a good one to follow.

In many workout routines, you follow a pretty standard pattern of one inhalation as you prepare to do a repetition, one exhalation as you do the repetition, and another inhalation as you prepare for the next rep.

However, handstand training (for the most part) doesn't involve repetitions and the normal pattern of inhaling and exhaling—instead, you are typically trying to hold a position for as long as you can while you attempt to maintain your balance.

This means that instead of that normal pattern, you'll focus on inhaling, and then a slow, steady, long exhale as you hold the position (and repeat that breathing pattern at the end of the exhale, if you're still able to hold the position).

That pattern of breathing serves two purposes. First, of course, it will help to keep you strong and steady while you're doing the exercise.

The second benefit is more mental. For people who are becoming familiar with handstand training, it can feel odd to be upside down and in the handstand position. If you focus on your breathing, however, that can go a long way toward taking your mind off of everything else and allowing you to find the strength and balance you need without thinking so much about it.

Now, I know I'm going to talk a lot about thinking about your handstand training, and how important it is to pay attention to what you're doing so that you can tweak your form, so it might sound weird when I say that you want to balance without thinking about it.

But there's an important distinction here—right after you've done (or attempted) a handstand, you should think about which direction you fell, and why, and try to figure out what you can do next time to correct for it.

Right before you do a handstand, you should think about what you've learned from your other attempts so you can use that while establishing your position, in order to make this handstand better.

But in the middle of the actual handstand, a lot of the time it's better if you drop the thinking and analysis to a minimum, focus on your breathing, and just try to balance instinctively.

It can be overwhelming to try to keep track of your hands, shoulders, feet, legs, and everything else all at once—which is why just thinking about steady, slow breathing, in and out, can often help you to stay focused as well as balanced.

JOINTS

When most people exercise nowadays, they tend to spend all of their time thinking about their muscles. However, to be strong and fit, you must also have strong joints, which a lot of athletes overlook. Many people fail to understand that, just as you can develop your muscles to be stronger and healthier, you can do the same with your joints.

In the ultra-controlled exercise environment that most people like to use today—with machines and gadgets that control your range of motion completely—your joints rarely deal with any kind of unexpected situation. However, the predictable environment created by those machines does not match up with the real world, which means that training your body—and your joints in particular—in this way will probably not prepare them for the real world, either.

That can lead to injury when you leave the gym and actually try to play a sport, or pick up something heavy, or do a cartwheel, or whatever.

Handstand training is different. It's unpredictable. You're trying to balance, which might mean tipping in one direction or another, or shifting your hand placement, or even tumbling out of the handstand if you can no longer hold it.

This can seem kind of scary if you're only used to exercising on machines, where nothing unpredictable ever happens, but it's also good training. It puts your joints and muscles into unfamiliar and unpredictable situations and forces them to react accordingly.

As long as you follow the progression in this book, your joints will have the chance to develop as they need to so that you can learn to hold a proper handstand.

Bear in mind that nothing is risk-free, and no matter how many precautions you take it is, of course, always possible to injure yourself doing this training or any other training, but the progression of exercises you will learn is intended to minimize that risk as much as is reasonably possible.

As you go through that progression, though, you might notice some discomfort here and there, during or after exercise. Discomfort can be perfectly safe and normal as your joints are exposed to new stresses and they learn to adapt.

However, that discomfort should fade. If it ever becomes pain, then you should stop what you're doing and make sure you're using proper form. If you still feel that pain after attempting the exercise again, you should go back and spend time doing some easier exercise that puts a little less stress on your joints.

Joints take more time than muscles to develop and strengthen, and you may find that you need to give them more time than you'd like. If you experience joint pain during a workout, then end your workout for the day and try again when the pain is gone, even if your muscles aren't tired yet.

Training to do handstands is an adjustment, so don't be surprised if you notice your body adjusting. Most of you probably won't need to give this a second thought, but some of you might.

I remember the day after one of my first extended handstand workouts I could hear an audible crackling sound when I moved my shoulders forward and back. It wasn't painful, or even uncomfortable, but it was definitely off-putting.

The next day, it was gone, and it never came back. Your body will adjust too, like mine did, though it might not be so noticeable.

Just go patiently through the progression, and if you run into any pain, drop back down to an easier exercise and work your way as slowly back up as you need to in order to stay pain-free.

WARMING UP

If you're seriously pursuing these handstand skills, you probably have enough experience with exercise to know that you need to warm up ahead of time.

That way, your blood will be flowing and your joints and muscles will be warm, which means you will both perform better during your workout, and be less likely to injure yourself during the workout.

Always be sure to warm up, and then stretch afterward. The order is important, because you will have much better results stretching muscles that are already warm.

You can have a decent warm up simply doing a few sets of 10-20 jumping jacks and toe touches, and then add a set or two of 10-20 pushups in there to get some of the muscles in your upper body working a little bit.

You don't quite need to be sweating, but you want to get your heart pumping and get mentally and physically ready for your handstand training. The more of these workouts you do, the more you'll get a sense of what exactly you need to do to feel 'warm.'

It's easy to forsake your warm-up in this or any other exercise routine. I don't recommend it. Always be sure to warm up.

STRETCHES

When you do any kind of workout, you should warm up and then stretch afterward. What we'll talk about in this chapter is not a full stretching routine, just one that is targeted toward what we'll be doing in your handstand work out.

First, do your warm up, as discussed in the previous chapter. Once you're warm, do any normal stretching routine that you're used to doing, and be sure to include these stretches for your triceps, shoulders, and hands:

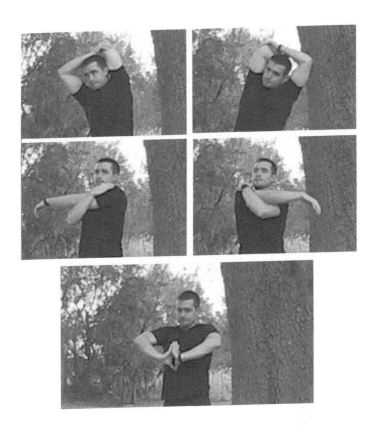

It's absolutely essential that you be sure to stretch your forearms and hands. In the last stretch pictured, you should apply gentle pressure to your fingertips as you lightly extend your arms. You should feel this motion stretching out your forearms. You can rotate your hands up or down while applying this pressure to shift the focus to different muscles in your forearm.

It should go without saying that the health and condition of your hands will be paramount to your success in your handstand training, and it's very easy to run into problems if you start off on the wrong foot by failing to stretch your hands.

THE EXERCISES

PUSHUPS

I almost wasn't going to include pushups as one of the exercises in here, because if you're attempting handstands then I would guess you're already proficient at these, but I suppose it makes sense to include them in the beginning.

Obviously, in order to do handstands, you're going to need some arm strength. It doesn't take exceptional upper body strength just to hold a handstand against a wall for a short time, but for some people (especially if you're on the heavier side, or if you don't have a lot of experience with exercise) the initial arm strength may be an issue. That's where the pushups come in.

On a basic level, the strength you will need to hold a handstand against a wall will come from your triceps and your shoulders, and even though the muscular focus is not exactly the same, you can build that kind of strength through pushups (not to mention the fact that pushups are just a good exercise, however basic they may be).

So, if you're a little rusty, or you feel a little unsure of your ability to support your full weight on your arms, you might want to begin working toward your goal of a free handstand by doing a few sets of pushups for a few workouts. You'll want to follow the pictures, and be sure to inhale as you go down, and exhale as you push up.

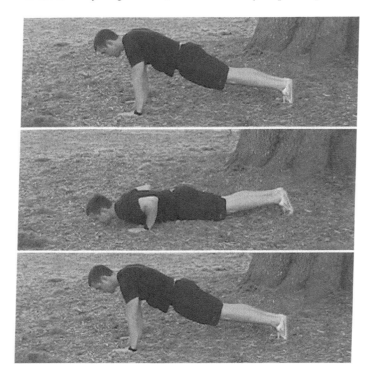

You should feel pretty good about your ability to hold a handstand against the wall if you can bang out 20 pushups, but really you should be able to even if you can just do 10 in good form. Like I said, it doesn't take a tremendous amount of upper body strength to do a wall handstand, and in the beginning the challenge is more about the mental and physical adjustment of being upside down than it is about being strong enough to hold the position.

If you feel that it's necessary, you might make your first workout (or your first few workouts) targeted toward the handstand about doing 3-5 sets of maybe 10-25 pushups (more pushups if you're on the lighter side, fewer if you're on the heavier side). If you can do that with no problem, then move right into the next exercise (Kick Ups). If not, you might want to keep at it until achieving those pushup numbers is pretty easy.

If this whole thing sounds way too basic and easy, don't worry about it and move right into the next exercise.

KICK UPS

This is basically just the first step of doing a wall handstand. It will become second nature before too long, but for now we want to focus specifically on what it takes to kick up against the wall and into a wall handstand.

Follow the sequence in the pictures: start on all fours, facing a wall, with your hands a little wider than shoulder-width apart, and your fingertips one to two feet away from the wall.

Next, plant one foot on the ground and raise the other into the air, as in picture 3. Gently and smoothly press off of your bottom foot hard enough that you are able to bring the top foot to the wall, then bring up your trailing foot to rest against the wall afterward. You are now holding a wall handstand.

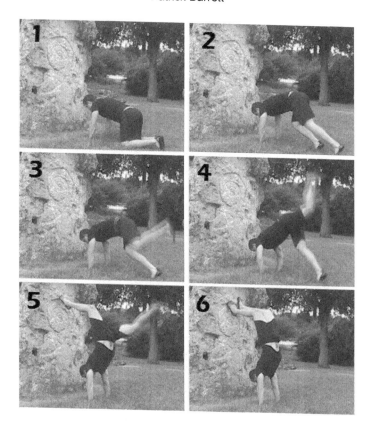

Some of you will nail this on your first try, but others will have trouble getting into position. That's fine; there are ways for you to ease into it. Remember these tips as you work on it:

1. Don't think so much about kicking up into the handstand that you forget to support your weight once you're in position. Keep you arms strongly extended, and be ready to support yourself in the handstand.

2. At first, kicking up a little too gently is better than doing it too forcefully—that way, you give yourself a chance to ease into the feeling of inverting yourself as you get into position. Just jump lightly off of the bottom foot, and try to bring your top foot up toward the wall. If you don't quite make it there, try again with a slightly stronger jump, and continue increasing the force of the jump until you make it over. That's much better than slamming yourself against the wall because you jumped as hard as you could (there's still a dent in the drywall at my parents' house from when I was showing an overzealous friend how to kick up back in high school).

Be patient, and spend the extra two minutes it takes to learn to kick up gently and smoothly—doing so will also create good habits for when you start to work on a real handstand.

3. Don't try to swing both legs up at the same time; if you do that, you'll come up all at once with far too much force. Learn to lead with one leg, and bringing the other up after it will be easy.

4. Once you're in a handstand, breathe deeply and slowly and stretch your whole body out; imagine you're standing on your tiptoes and trying to reach above your head as high as you can. Focus on your breathing, and hold that position.

Side Note: In picture 6, my legs are bent at about 90 degrees, simply because of how far I am from the wall. If your fingertips are more in the one-foot-from-the-wall range, you'll be able to hold the wall handstand with straighter legs. Either is fine at this point.

5. To get down, just do the reverse—press lightly off the wall with (what was) your top foot, and bring your bottom foot back down to the floor, followed by your top foot.

That's all it takes. Again, once you get it down this part will be incredibly easy, but you need to get the muscle memory down in the beginning, and you need to develop the body awareness associated with going from being upright to being upside down.

Once you've successfully done it two or three times in a row, you'll do sets of these, kicking up, holding for a second or two, and then coming back down, so that you are thoroughly comfortable with the movement.

WALL HANDSTANDS

The wall handstand is a simple enough exercise once you've mastered the kick up; you will simply hold the up position for as long as you can do it correctly. There are a few things that you'll want to keep in mind as you're doing these handstands, however.

In the beginning, do the handstands with your fingertips around one to two feet from the wall. This distance makes it easy for you to lean against the wall for support. However, as you become more comfortable, move your hands closer, until you can kick up comfortably with your fingertips within six inches of the wall, and then within three. The closer your hands get to the wall, the more your weight will be above your hands, as opposed to against the wall. This will more closely approximate the feeling of doing an actual handstand.

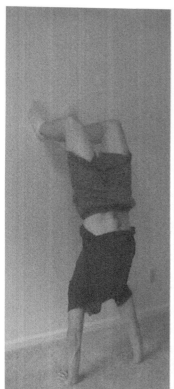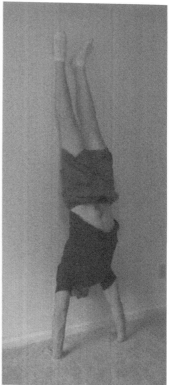

The first picture shows a handstand with fingertips about 18 inches from the wall. The greater distance is the reason for the bent legs. This position allows you to lean more heavily against the wall, and is easier to hold for most beginners.

The second picture shows a handstand with fingertips three or four inches from the wall—as you can see, being closer to the wall means your legs will be straighter. Because you are right up against the wall, more of your weight will be directly over your hands, which will force you to rely less on the wall and more on your own strength.

The next exercise you do will require you to have your fingertips only a few inches from the wall, so work on getting comfortable with that—the closer your hands are to the wall, the more you will begin to feel what it's like to hold a free handstand.

While you are holding the handstand, don't just lean your whole body against the wall like dead weight. Remember that your goal is to do a handstand without the wall's help. Try to support yourself as much as possible on your own hands, and imagine the feeling of holding the position without the wall's help. Lean lightly, as much as you need to, but bear in mind that your purpose is to get to the point that you won't need to lean at all.

Focus on deep, slow breathing, and remember to extend and stretch your body. When you come down, don't collapse off the wall, but do it in as much control as you can—it will help you to develop the instincts you need to hold an actual handstand.

PUSHAWAYS

These are a big step toward being able to do a handstand.

Kick into a wall handstand with your fingertips around three inches away from the wall. Hold the position firmly, extend yourself, and feel as much of your weight as possible on your hands. Keep your legs straight.

Now, smoothly and firmly apply downward pressure with your fingers. If you're not leaning too hard on the wall, you should start to feel your legs push away from the wall. Your goal is to push hard enough that your legs come off the wall entirely, and you hold a handstand for a second or two (or longer, if you can). If you don't move at first, concentrate on applying pressure with your fingertips in particular.

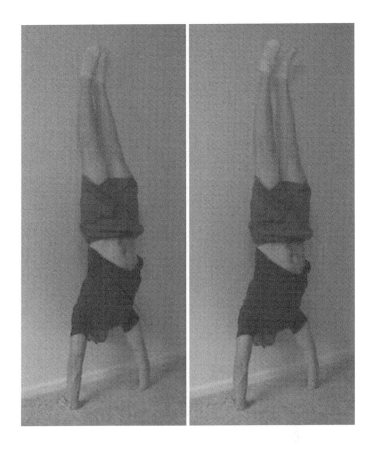

As you can see in the picture, there is not an enormous visual difference between the first picture and the second picture—but there is a huge difference for you, because in the first position you are doing a handstand against the wall, and in the second position (if you can hold it), you have pushed your feet away from the wall, and you are doing a brief free handstand.

If you are unable to push off from the wall at all, you may need to come down, and kick back up with your fingertips closer to the wall—the closer your fingertips are to the wall, the easier it will be to push off from the wall (because you're closer to being upright), and the farther away they are, the harder it will be (because you're leaning on the wall a lot more). If your fingertips are already very close to the wall, work on putting more of your own weight above your hands (and less leaning against the wall), and keep trying to push down with your fingers (especially your fingertips if you're having trouble).

You will learn a lot from doing this exercise, because it's the first time you'll really be holding a free handstand without any help from a wall (even if only for a second). After pushing off from the wall, try to hold your balance as long as you can. You want to rely primarily on your hands and fingers to keep your balance, not by trying to swing your legs in one direction or the other—so be sure to keep your whole body straight and extended, and balance by applying pressure to your fingers, or to the heels of your hands (more on that in later chapters).

Once you lose your balance, you'll either fall back down to the ground, or you'll fall against the wall. If you fall down to the ground, kick back up and try again. If you fall back against the wall, ready yourself to push away again, and try to hold for a second or two longer.

Pay attention to which way you tend to fall, and try to correct for it—but don't get too frustrated. You need to develop the balance, which will take practice, but you also have to have strong hands and fingers to hold a handstand, and developing that strength takes a little time. Keep at it, and you'll see improvements from workout to workout.

As you start to get better at this, move your fingertips a little farther from the wall (remember, the farther your fingertips, the harder it will be to push off). When you really get the hang of it, try to use pressure from your fingertips as you kick up to slow, or even stop yourself before your feet even touch the wall. When your fingers are strong enough to do that, you're getting close to being able to hold a real handstand.

HANDWALKING

Handwalking is fun. It's not absolutely necessary, but if you've got the space and the inclination to do it, it can be a great way to develop better strength and balance in the handstand.

The premise is simple. Find an open space where you're comfortable falling down, and kick up into a handstand. As you start to fall forward, throw a hand out to catch yourself, then follow with the other hand, and so forth. Keep leaning forward a little, and keep putting your hands out to catch yourself, until you can't anymore. At that point you'll probably fall down, and you can catch your breath and try again.

Most people like to do this on grass, and you should probably do it there to avoid any hard falls. To follow the progression in the picture, look down the first column of images in sequence, and then down the second column.

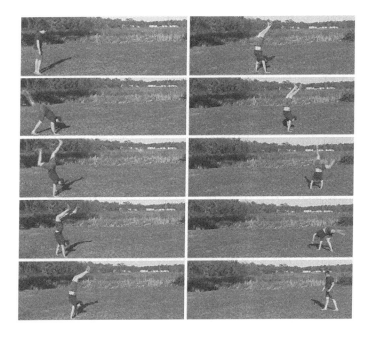

As you can see in the picture, you'll start from standing, and then lean down and kick up at the same time. You can see that you will need to extend your legs far forward, because you need to lean forward to go forward—and the farther you lean, the faster you'll need to walk to keep up with your weight. There are many ways to end a handwalk, but most of them in the beginning amount to semi-controlled falling down.

You can see in this sequence in the 8th, 9th, and 10th pictures (middle to bottom of the second column) that one way to 'dismount' is to place a hand straight out ahead of you so you turn 90 degrees to one side, and then sort of 'cartwheel' out of it.

At first it will be a struggle to take two steps, but you might be surprised how far you can go. Handwalking doesn't really require much balance—you're kind of falling slightly forward, or to one side or the other, the whole time, and constantly moving and adjusting, so even if you can't hold a free handstand yet, you might be able to handwalk farther than you would have expected. It's sort of like how balancing on a bicycle is difficult if the bike is standing still in one place, but easy when that same bike is rolling forward.

Also, because you're so absorbed in trying to stay up, you don't realize how hard you're working, and you can make it a pretty strenuous workout while enjoying yourself.

Once you get a little better, and you can start trying for distance, it can be very helpful for developing balance, because you'll have to learn to stay upright as your hands, arms, back, and shoulders start to fatigue. Once you get better at balancing with tired hands at the end of a handwalk, it gets much easier with fresh hands during a handstand.

Like I said, you don't need to do any handwalking in order to learn to hold a handstand. If you don't feel comfortable with it, or if you don't have a safe place to do it, don't worry about it, and move on to the next section.

HANDSTAND

If you've spent enough time working on the pushaway that you can start to hold a solid handstand without the support of the wall, then you should start to work on the real thing.

The first big change will be in the way you kick up. Before, you would get down on all fours, and then kick up against the wall.

Now, you will go from standing directly into the handstand as pictured, without getting down on all fours. I'll explain the movement briefly, and then we'll go back over it and look at the details.

Take a look at the pictures:

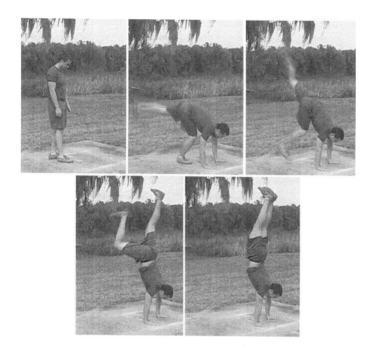

Stand in a clear, flat, open area, with one foot slightly behind the other. Lean down, and place your hands on the floor. As you put your hands down, bring your lead foot up behind you. As you shift your weight down onto your hands, bring your trailing foot up beside your lead foot. Hold the handstand for as long as you can.

Now we'll look at each step in more detail:

You'll be standing in a flat, open space. There's an important thing to consider about where you choose to do your handstand—you may want to pick a grassy area, so it's softer if you fall down. A softer fall is nice, but it's actually a lot harder to balance on soft terrain. When you push your fingertips into soft ground to try to balance, the ground will give, and you won't get the resistance you need, which will make you push harder, and overcorrect.

It's much easier to find stable balance on a hard surface. This makes for a harder fall, if you do fall, but by now you should have enough experience coming down out of a handstand that you won't hurt yourself. It doesn't have to be asphalt or bare concrete; linoleum or short carpet can be fine, but you'll probably need something at least that firm, as opposed to grass or dirt.

Place one foot behind the other—the rear foot will be the foot you lead with, and the other foot will be the last to leave the ground as you go up into your handstand.

When you bend down, let your arms hang loosely so that your hands touch the ground directly below your shoulders. If you reach forward as you lean down, you'll have a hard time kicking hard enough to get your weight above your hands. If you bring your hands in too close to your feet, you'll probably kick too hard and flip over. Just let your arms hang naturally as you bend down, so that your hands come down directly below your shoulder, which is where they need to be for optimal balance.

Spread your fingers a little bit; this will help to create a stable base on the ground, and give your fingers leverage to support you.

By the time your hands touch down, your leading leg should be straight out behind you. Keep it moving in one steady motion until it is straight above you. As that leg comes up and your weight shifts solidly onto your hands, bring up your trailing leg to join your lead leg.

This is a hugely important part of doing a handstand—do not kick both legs up together. Bringing up one leg, and then the other, makes a huge difference in your ability to balance. To the observer in real time, there's probably less than a second between the one leg coming up and the second leg coming up, but it makes a huge difference for the guy doing the handstand.

Think about it: your legs are pretty heavy, and they're the farthest part of you from your hands. Which direction they're swinging in, or where they're leaning, pretty much determines whether you're going to balance in a handstand or fall over. You need a good foundation with hand strength, to be sure, but body awareness and control of your legs is every bit as important.

If you kick both legs up at once, you've got very little control. Either you kicked them up with the perfect amount of force (very unlikely), or you kicked too hard or too soft, which means you'll end up falling over, even if you manage to hang there for a second or two.

Separating them into a leading leg and a trailing leg means you can get most of your weight up there with the first leg, and then depending on where you are with that leg, you can adjust the way your second leg comes in. If the first leg comes in too fast, you can bring the second leg in just a bit more slowly. If your first leg kicks out to one side, your second leg can compensate. Basically, leading with one leg, then following right after with the other, gives you two chances to get your balance right, instead of just one.

This might not make much sense as you read it, but you'll really see what I mean once you start practicing for the handstand.

It's crucial that you understand how important your legs are for balance when it comes to the handstand. I like to do at least one handstand every time I exercise, whether I'm focusing on pressing movements, or pulling movements, or my lower body, or whatever I'm doing. Do you know when it's hardest to do a good handstand? Not after a hard pressing workout, when I've been doing dips and pushups and various presses, and not after a hard pulling workout, when my hands are worn out from being on the pull up bar.

The hardest time by far to do a good handstand is after a lower body workout, because it's so much harder to be precise with those little adjustments of your legs, and also because the tightness in your legs after a lower body workout changes the way you kick up, which throws off your balance.

If your hands or your arms are worn out, that's not such a big deal. Tired legs make all the difference, which you'll see if you pay attention when you start working on the handstand.

Once I'm up in a handstand, I like to focus on looking at the ground and taking deep breaths, in and out. Try to keep your weight balanced right in the center of your palm. If you start to tip forward, push your fingers flat into the ground to compensate. If you start to tip a lot, push with your fingertips. If you start to tip backward, pick your hand up and drive the heel of your hand into the ground.

Try this exercise to understand the best way to balance with your hand. Stand barefoot on a hard, flat surface. Lean forward, just slightly. Do you feel how you put pressure into the forward part of your foot? Now lean forward more. Notice how the pressure shifts quickly from the front of your foot out to the tips of your toes—you get better leverage from the tips of your toes, just like you get better leverage from the tips of your fingers. That's why if you want to correct just a little bit, you should push down evenly along the length of your whole finger, but if you're tipping forward more drastically, you need to use the fingertips to save your handstand.

Let's go back to standing barefoot. Now, lean back a little bit. Do you notice how you pick your feet up, and drive your weight down into your heels to keep from falling backward? Again, it's just the same if you find yourself falling backwards in the handstand—pick your hand up, and drive the weight down into the heel of your hand.

Remember that your hands are operating like feet, so if you keep having one problem or another, try to diagnose the issue by standing barefoot, leaning one way or another, and seeing how you correct, and then seeing how you can apply that during a handstand.

You want your weight balanced basically in the center of your palm. Ideally, you shouldn't need any compensating pressure through your fingers, or from the heel of your hand to stay upright, just that weight balanced right in the middle of your palm.

When you feel the weight start to slide forward, apply pressure to your fingers to move it back where it belongs. When you feel it start to slide back, pick your hand up and drive down the weight through the heel of your hand to shift your balance back. In the beginning you will probably overcorrect and end up falling in the opposite direction from where you were falling before you corrected, but that's a necessary part of the process you have to go through before you get the right instincts.

Ideally, once you've gone through all of that and you have a better idea of how to keep your balance, you want to keep things under control so you can use small adjustments to stay balanced without overcorrecting.

When you come down from the handstand, try to do it under your own power. Instead of just falling to one side or the other, or your arms giving out, deliberately bring down your trailing foot, and then your lead foot, and stand back up. This reinforces the good habit of staying in control throughout your entire handstand, all the way until you return to standing.

TRAINING FOR THE FREE HANDSTAND

Because of the nature of handstand training—because it's as much about developing a skill as it is about building physical strength—the schedule you follow will tend to be a little different from what you follow during normal strength training.

If you want to see real progress in your handstand training, I would recommend that you work on it at least three times a week for at least a half an hour per workout. In the beginning, as your body adjusts to this mode of exercise, I wouldn't go too far beyond that, but once you're several weeks in and you start to be comfortable with your handstand training, you can start to work on it more often than that.

You might decide to work on it a lot more than that—personally, I like to do at least one handstand a day to stay in practice, with more extended workouts two to four times a week, depending on whatever else I'm working on.

In the beginning, when you're still learning how to hold a free handstand, follow this progression (always remember to warm up and stretch before each workout):

Phase 1
Do 3-5 wall handstands, with 1-2 minutes of rest in between. Hold each handstand for as long you can with proper form. For extra work, do 1-3 sets of kick ups afterwards (again, continue each set for as long as you can kick up properly). Get more comfortable moving your fingertips closer to the wall from workout to workout, until they are just a few inches from the wall.

Once you can comfortably hold a wall handstand (with your fingertips around three inches from the wall) for a minute, move on to the next phase, when you focus on getting comfortable with the free handstand.

Phase 2
Work on the handstand pushaways, and try to hold the free handstand for as long as you can each time you push away. If you fall back against the wall, take a second to get ready and then attempt to push away again. If you fall to the ground, take a breath, wait 30 seconds or a minute if you need to, and kick back up and try again. You might need a break for a minute or two here or there depending on how long you work on this. Work on these for as long as they still feel productive—probably anywhere from 5 to 20 minutes.

Alternately, you can spend some workouts focused on handwalking. Just find a flat, open area, kick up, try to walk for as long as you can, rest a minute or so, and try again. As with the pushaways, around 5-20 minutes should be good, just until you feel like you're tired enough that your form is suffering.

At some point your hands, arms, or shoulders will start to get tired, you will feel like you're getting worse instead of better. Stop doing the handstand pushaways or handwalking; if you want a little bit more of workout, you can do another 1-3 handstands against a wall, but you should be pretty much done with your handstands at that point.

Once you can push away from the wall and hold what feels like an almost solid handstand for a few seconds, it's time to move into the next phase.

Phase 3
Find a flat, open space, and start working on free handstands. At this point, you can basically work on them for as long it feels productive—as before, there will come a point when your hands, or your shoulders, or your arms will start to get worn out, and your attempts will become less and less successful.

You always want to stop if you run into any joint pain, but once you've got the basics down, feel free to keep trying as long as you feel like it's productive—in other words, if you're so worn out that you keep dropping right down the second you kick up, you should probably call it a day. However, if you've been working for a while but you still feel like you're making progress, then feel free to keep going.

When you're in phase three, make sure that you train intelligently. Don't just kick up over and over again and keep falling down in the same direction. Pay attention when you fall, think about why it happened, and correct it for the next time—more often than not, your hands are probably in the wrong position, or you're kicking up one of your legs too hard or soft, or in the wrong direction. You could work on free handstands for an hour without stopping to correct your mistakes, and wouldn't be as productive as five minutes of actively trying to diagnose and fix your problems.

Refer back to the section on Free Handstands under exercises so you know what to look out for—how to kick up properly, where to drop your hands, and so on. In the beginning, you might be doing several things wrong. Try to pinpoint one, work on solving it, and then move on to the next one.

Just be sure to take a second between attempts to think about the little adjustments you might want to make on your next try.

Once you can reliably kick up into a handstand, hold it, and come down in control, you're really out of phase 3 and into normal handstand training. You can mix doing free handstands into your normal upper body routine.

One simple way is to do 3-5 handstands, each for as long as you can, with a couple of minutes' rest in between. You can also start training to do handstand pushups, which you can read about in the next chapters.

PIKE PUSHUPS

The pike pushup is a modified pushup. It's a great way to start building the strength and body awareness you need to do handstand pushups, whether they are against a wall, or free standing. This type of pushup moves the muscular focus of the movement from your chest and arms to your shoulders and arms, and uses a range of motion which is similar to the range of motion in a handstand pushup.

There are two basic ways to do a pike pushup. Take a look at the pictures:

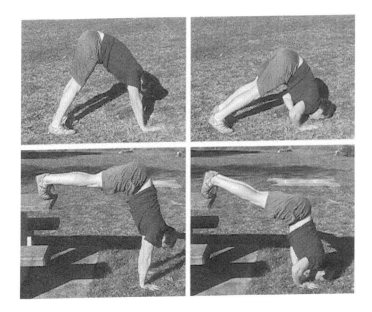

The first is to bend at your waist, keep your legs straight, and put your hands on the ground 2 to 3 feet in front of your feet. Keep your back as flat as you can (this requires a little bit of flexibility to really do it well, but even if you're not too flexible it can be very helpful). Do pushups by bringing your nose to the floor, and then pushing back up to the starting position. As always, inhale on your way down, and exhale on your way back up.

The other way to do them is basically the same, but you elevate your feet. You can put your feet on anything that won't fall over easily—a stack of mats, the edge of a bed, a balance ball. The idea is just to raise yourself up and get your hips—and more of your weight—above your hands. This obviously makes the movement more difficult, and more like a handstand pushup.

You will probably be surprised at how difficult these can be when you do them right. You should feel it in your triceps and the tops of your shoulders. If you can't go all the way down in the beginning, go down as far as you can, and then push back up. Work on going down a little farther, and a little farther each time until you can go the whole way.

WALL HANDSTAND PUSHUPS

Handstand pushups are a phenomenal way to build upper body strength. Doing them without the support of a wall is much more difficult—and much more impressive—but realistically, you'll be able to get in a lot more reps, and build more strength in your arms and shoulders, when you do them against a wall.

Handstand pushups against a wall are pretty self-explanatory. As you see in the pictures, you kick up into a wall handstand with fingertips 3 to 6 inches from the wall, lower yourself until your nose touches the floor, and then press back up. Repeat until you can't do them any more.

If you've been doing a lot of work with handstands and pike pushups, you might be able to go all the way down and back up on your first try. If that's the case, then do sets of one, or two, or however many you can, and work on doing more reps as you would with any other exercise. However, if you can't do a full rep in proper form, there

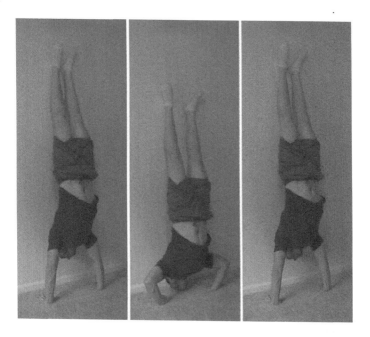

are two basic ways you're going to work on it: partial reps, and negatives. We'll look at partial reps first.

If you've been doing a lot of work with handstands and pike pushups, you might be able to go all the way down and back up on your first try. If that's the case, then do sets of one, or two, or however many you can, and work on doing more reps as you would with any other exercise. However, if you can't do a full rep in proper form, there are two basic ways you're going to work on it: partial reps, and negatives. We'll look at partial reps first.

Partial reps are simple. If you can't go all the way down and come back, go down as far as you can, while still being able to come back up. Start out by going down an inch or so (you should have no problem coming up from that if you've been doing any work with the pike pushups). Then go down a little more than an inch, and a little more, and so on. Within a few reps you should be able to find a sticking point you can't go past and come back up from.

Do as many reps as you can, as deep into that sticking point as you can, while still coming back up. Rest a couple of minutes, and repeat for 3-5 sets, or as long as you feel like you're being productive. After a few workouts, you'll notice yourself being able to get lower and lower, until you can touch your nose to the floor.

The other way to get there is through negatives. Just lower yourself in as much control as you can until you're all the way the bottom. Then push your feet off the wall so you come down from the handstand, kick back up, and do another negative. You can take two approaches—do the negatives as slowly as possible, to make each negative as difficult as possible, or do them as quickly as you can while maintaining control, then kick back up and do more, so you get in as many total reps as you can. Both can work, and you will probably want to do a mix in your workouts to keep things interesting and effective.

After a few workouts with partial reps and negative reps, you should see a big increase in your range of motion until you are able to perform full range handstand pushups against a wall.

HANDSTAND PUSHUPS

Handstand pushups, done without assistance from a wall, are one of the more impressive feats of balance and upper body strength in most people's eyes, and rightly so. Training for them is relatively simple, especially if you've mastered everything we've discussed so far in this book.

If you can hold a free handstand comfortably, and you can do handstand pushups while leaning against a wall, you can start to work on putting the two together. The process is basically the same as training for the handstand pushups with a wall, and you'll be using partial reps and negatives again, in much the same way, with the same progression.

When I do handstand pushups, I like to come all the way down until my nose touches the floor—as far as I can go with hands on the floor. That's going to mean your head coming forward a little bit, which will mean you legs leaning back a little to compensate (as you can see). Expect this movement, and be ready to compensate for it, on the way down as well as on the way up.

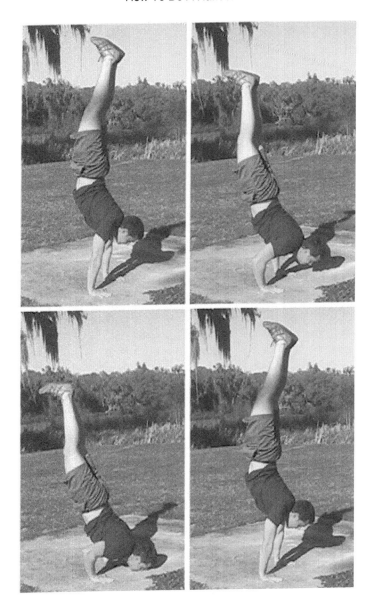

Just as when you hold a handstand, you want to keep your balance in the middle of your palm as you go down and press back up. Keeping balance on your way down and up will go a long way toward making the movement possible.

A lot of people who have the strength to complete this movement are unable to because they can't keep their balance in check on the way down, and they think they can muscle through it. Think about it—if you're trying to press up, but you're losing your balance forward, you're going to start pressing down hard on your fingers to keep your balance. Now all that strength you're exerting through your arms and shoulders isn't lifting your body up, it's directed through your fingers, and making you lean back.

Now you're overcorrecting, and you're going to fall down. Doing full negatives is especially important when training for the handstand pushup, not just to build the strength you need, but to learn to keep your balance as you bend your arms. That way, when you press up to lift yourself back up, the force of your movement will be directed into your palm, and will actually be productive, and lift you up.

Many people who don't take the time to get the balance right will find themselves feeling like it's impossible to lift themselves from the down position—then for a moment they'll catch their balance just right and shoot up, because they were finally directing the force through the palms of their hands, instead of losing it into their fingertips as they struggled for balance.

Like much of these descriptions, this will all make more sense as you train for this movement, and you may find that once you get the hang of it, you'll find your own little variation that works best for you.

Work on it little by little. In the beginning, just try to drop down an inch or so, to get yourself used to the idea of keeping your balance as you move. Stick with partial reps in the beginning to develop that sense of balance, and only after you can go down and up for a few inches should you start to try the negatives all the way down. Then mix both of them into your workout, continuing to develop both strength and balance until you can lower your nose to the floor and press all the way up for a complete handstand pushup.

GENERAL COMMENTS ON
HANDSTAND TRAINING

In the beginning, you will work just to be able to do these exercises at all. While you do that, use the progressions and advice in "Training For The Free Handstand," and the descriptions of the pushup exercises. However, once you are able to do all of these things, you will want to incorporate them into your general workout routine.

Some people are only interested in being able to do handstands, and are not so interested in the pushups. Simple handstand training is easy to fit into a person's schedule or workout routine. It can be as easy as doing one handstand a day, and holding it for as long as you can. Alternatively, you can hold 3-5 handstands with a few minutes rest in between, 2-5 times a week or so.

If you feel able to do more, and you aren't experiencing any joint pain or anything, feel free to do more—the strenuousness of handstand training varies to some degree with your size and fitness level, but generally speaking, if you want to do more, do more. If you like handwalking, it can also be beneficial to walk along a certain path, or a certain distance, on a regular basis.

If you are also interested in the pushups, you probably want to use a more structured approach. As a general rule, when you structure handstand pushup workouts, you want to do free standing exercises before you do anything against a wall, and within those two groups you want to do pressing exercises before you do handstands.

In other words, you might follow a routine like this (after warming up and stretching of course):

1. Work on handstand pushups for 5 or 10 minutes.

2. Do a couple of handstands for as long as you can hold them.

3. Do a few sets of handstand pushups against a wall.

4. Finish with 3 sets of pike pushups.

Let's look at that routine in slightly more detail.

Often, it's less common to say "Do three sets of 2 handstand pushups" and more common to say "work on handstand pushups for a certain amount of time." They are a little unpredictable for most people, even after you become comfortable with them, and for the most part, when you attempt them, you're just trying to do as many as you can in good form. You may lose your balance after one during your first attempt, then wait a minute or two and crank out five good ones.

I find it's best to warm up, try to do a few handstand pushups, wait a minute or so, try again, and repeat until your arms get fatigued, you feel like you're no longer being productive, and you're ready to move to an easier exercise—could be five minutes, could be 45 minutes. Your reps, and your level of mastery, will increase as you spend more time on your hands.

If you're a competitive gymnast or a dancer or another dedicated person, you probably want to strive for a higher level of discipline, and I applaud that. However, if you're just a 'regular guy' training to do handstands—as most people who read this book are—I think it helps to maintain the attitude described in the previous paragraph.

After handstand pushup training, you move to handstands, which should be a bit more predictable. The handstands will be more challenging now that you're fatigued from the pushups, so you'll get a better workout. I like to do 1-3 handstands with a couple of minutes in between, but you can vary it how you like, or move straight to the next part.

Once you're done with free handstands, you can move to the wall to do some handstand pushups. A lot of times it's your ability to balance that gives out before your upper body with the handstand pushups, so doing a few sets against a wall can help make sure that your arms and shoulders are getting in the hard work they need to get stronger. I like to do 1-3 sets of as many as I can.

If you still want more, you can work in some pike pushups at the end of that, and of course if you'd like to finish with wall handstands you can do that too, although often once people can do free handstands they don't do much more work with wall handstands.

That will give you a nice, complete handstand pushup routine. You can change the length of this routine a good deal depending on how many sets and attempts of each thing you do. If you're working this in to a larger upper body pressing routine, you might make it a lot shorter; if this is your entire pressing routine, you can make it longer. Just decide how much of a priority you want to make this, and plan accordingly.

A NOTE ON FORM

There are people who do handstands as part of a competition, and there are people who do them primarily for exercise. Now, the people who do them for a competition (gymnasts, primarily) also do them for exercise, but their goal in the end is to be able to perform handstands and have them judged to be technically correct.

I am not a competitive gymnast. I am not trained to do handstands like a competitive gymnast should. In fact, I'm not trained in any way; what I've learned has been almost exclusively through trial and error.

I think gymnastics is awesome, don't get me wrong, I just want to make it clear that I am not any kind of authority on what it means to do a handstand in a way that a judge will approve of.

One thing that I've learned is that almost everybody has their definition of what a 'correct' or 'incorrect' version of an exercise is. Sometimes it's an important distinction—

sometimes the correct version can be beneficial while the incorrect version can lead to joint issues or injuries down the line.

However, I've found that most discussion over the correctness or incorrectness of a handstand is unnecessary at best. For the most part, if a person has his hands on the ground instead of his feet, it's a good bet that whatever he's doing is some kind of handstand.

Within the term "handstand" there is a world of variation. Some handstands rely more on strength; some rely more on balance—to that end, some people make a distinction between a "handstand" and a "handbalance." Some are rigid and straight, and some have more of a "graceful arch" to them. There have been famous strongmen and athletes whose handstands fit into both categories, and one isn't more of a handstand than the other.

Whether or not something is a handstand is fairly obvious. If you're standing on your hands, and if doing it doesn't result in any kind of joint pain or back pain, it's probably a good handstand in my book. My advice to you is that unless you're doing handstands as some part of a competition (in which case you should talk to your coach, and ignore me), leave the squabbling to other people. Instead of commenting on whether someone else's handstand is a "real" handstand, or listening to them to find out if yours is "real," spend some more time training, or doing something enjoyable. There are more important things to worry about.

This question gets a little more interesting when it comes to handstand pushups. With handstands, you are holding a static position. With a handstand pushup, you are going through a range of motion, and as a general rule it is always best to follow completely through a range of motion, and not stop at some arbitrary point.

You learned to do partial reps on some exercises earlier, but that can be fine as long as you increase to the full range of motion over time, instead of always doing partial reps.

So let's look at the handstand pushup. We went through the training you need to be able to lower yourself until your nose touches the floor, and then press back up. That's a full range of motion, right?

Well, yes and no. It's a full range of motion in that you're going all the way down as far you can go, and you're pushing back up all the way. However, what stops you on your way down is not your joints or muscles, it's the floor. In other words, if there were a big hole in the floor beneath your face, you could go down farther, for a more complete range of motion.

Serious gymnasts and athletes will use parallettes (mini horizontal bars) or specially designed canes or platforms to raise themselves up off the ground so they can lower themselves all the way down until their shoulders rest on their hands, and their heads are well below their hands. This is a true full range of motion for the handstand pushup.

Working up to that requires buying or building equipment, and putting yourself into a slightly more precarious physical position than the training we've talked about so far. If you'd like to pursue that, the progressions are fairly obvious (an extension of the partial reps and negatives we already talked about). Use a spotter and, ideally, an experienced coach of some kind.

A good, inexpensive compromise can be to continue all the training as we've already discussed it, but to do your wall handstand pushups with your hands up on matching, sturdy step stools or low chairs—again, use the negatives and partial reps to expand your range of motion. You'll be in a stable environment, with the wall to keep you up, and your elevated hands will allow you to go down even farther than you were previously.

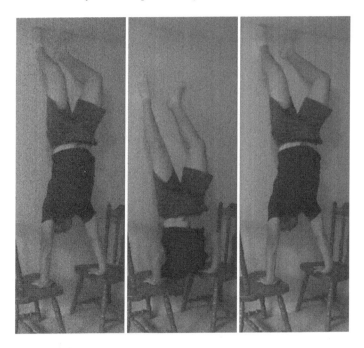

Experiment with placing your fingertips anywhere from 3-9 inches from the wall to find a comfortable position.

Kicking up into a handstand on chairs or stools is a little bit precarious at first; depending on how high they are, you may need to plant one foot on the edge of one of the chairs in order to get into position.

Learn this motion the way you learned how to kick up in the first place, by using small movements that get progressively larger and more forceful until you learn how much force you need to get up into your handstand.

NUTRITION

Like many types of "skill" oriented training, learning how to do handstands will require effective recovery between workouts. That means that your body will have to repair and strengthen muscle and joint tissues as you go through your training.

If your body is going to repair itself, it's going to need the proper materials. That's where your diet comes in.

The whole point of your training is to force your body to go through that strengthening and repairing process, so if you're not going to eat properly and give your body the nutrients it needs, then to some extent you're just wasting your time.

I'm not going to attempt to cover all of human nutrition in this one chapter. It's not possible, and it's not necessary. But you do need to have a basic understanding of this concept. If you do your training, but all you consume is beer, pizza, and candy bars, don't be surprised when you never seem to go anywhere.

That's a little bit of an extreme example, but the fact is that many people, even those who are pretty well convinced that they eat the "right" kinds of foods, are not giving their bodies what they really need to repair and recover optimally.

I've written a full book on this subject called The Natural Diet , and if you're interested in nutrition, then I definitely recommend that you take a look at it. It presents an approach to the question of human nutrition that's very different from, and really much simpler than, most of what else you'll find out there—and you'll certainly learn a thing or two you never knew before.

Even if you don't decide to read that book, there are a few basic mistakes we want to avoid, especially in the middle of something like handstand training that requires your body to repair muscles and joints as it adjusts to these new movements.

The first thing might be the most important—eat fat. Consuming healthy fat is absolutely critical to being a healthy person, particularly when your body is working to repair and maintain joint tissues.

When I say fat, I'm not talking about "vegetable oil" (AKA soy oil) or canola oil. I mean butter, olive oil, peanut oil, coconut oil—any minimally processed oil that still has an appetizing odor and flavor.

To make a long story short, fats that have no odor or flavor have gone through a lot of processing and the nutrients contained in them are severely damaged. You do not want to put these things in your body.

Avoid fats and oils that are heavily processed and/or have no odor or flavor. This includes any kind of margarine, "spreads," or bottled soy oil or canola oil. Instead, pick fats with only ONE ingredient that smell and test like food, such as real butter, peanut oil, olive oil, coconut oil, or palm oil, for example.

Next, eat fresh fruit. Fresh means it's not packed into a can, or floating in syrup, or juiced and pasteurized and put into a bottle—it's just a fresh piece of fruit from the produce section that hasn't been heated or processed. It's possibly the perfect fuel for your body, and it's something you absolutely must eat several times each day, without exception.

Last, avoid food additives whenever possible. There are many dozens of such additives that you might find in any number of foods, and some are much worse than others, but you don't need to spend all that time learning which one is which if you don't want to. Just avoid all of them. The bottom line is that although they are tested in a limited way so that they can be certified and put into foods, some of them are still very bad news, and nobody is quite sure what happens when you eat all of them together.

Avoid them. At best they just sort of get in the way of the normal processes that your body tries to do on a daily basis, and at worse they can directly cause some serious problems, involving stomach upset, headaches, or worse. You can avoid the whole issue by eating wholesome foods with ingredients that you recognize.

Maintaining an optimal diet can have a huge positive effect on your training and your general well-being on a day-to-day basis. If this is something you're interested in, I recommend picking up a copy of my book, The Natural Diet . Even if you don't decide to read that book, sticking to these simple tips covered in this chapter will still do you a lot of good and keep you on track with your training.

CONCLUSION

Now you know everything you need to know to be able to hold a free handstand for a minute or more, or to do a free standing handstand pushup, or to walk on your hands, or perform a number of other skills.

A huge part of your success, though, will come from developing the muscle memory and intuitive balance that is critical in holding a handstand. You can only get there through consistent repetition and intelligent practice of these exercises.

If you tend to fall out of any of these exercises, try to pay attention to the direction in which you fall. Figure out what you can do with your hands, or your legs, or your head, or whichever part of your body is necessary to correct for that tendency.

Being smart and paying attention will increase the quality of the time you spend training to do handstands, and doing a moderate to high volume of high quality training will give you results that you will be very happy with.

However, simply drilling the same exact thing over and over again, without stopping and thinking about what exactly isn't working, won't get you very far. Neither will reading this book, practicing minimally, and thinking too much about the "theory" behind what you're doing instead of putting in the time so that your body can start to feel, intuitively, the right way to balance.

You've got to spend the time doing the training, and you've got to pay attention to what you're doing—to what's working, and to what isn't. If you won't do that, it doesn't matter how many handstand training books you read.

Having said all that, I'm definitely excited that you've chosen to pursue this skill. Doing handstands is without a doubt one of my favorite types of training, both because it builds strength in your hands, shoulders, abs, and back, and also because it develops your overall sense of balance.

Of course, doing handstands is also just fun, and really satisfying—much more so than any exercise I've ever done on a weight machine.

Becoming proficient at doing handstands takes some time and effort, but it is well worth it. Stick to the exercises, train hard, and give your body the food and rest it needs to recover afterward. You'll be glad you did.

OTHER BOOKS BY PATRICK BARRETT

Natural Exercise: Basic Bodyweight Training and Calisthenics for Strength and Weight-Loss

The Natural Diet: Simple Nutritional Advice For Optimal Health In The Modern World

One Arm Pull Up: Bodyweight Training And Exercise Program For One Arm Pull Ups And Chin Ups

ABOUT THE AUTHOR

Patrick Barrett has been interested in exercise ever since he started to lift weights with his dad and older brothers as a kid. He participated in a half-dozen organized sports (most notably inline hockey and high school wrestling) until a neck injury during a wrestling match in his junior year prevented him from playing further in any contact sports.

After the injury, he developed an interest in pursuing strength and balance, particularly through bodyweight and self-taught gymnastic-type exercises.

Patrick has always loved both cooking and eating food. Unsatisfied with the confusing and often contradictory nutritional advice offered by mainstream sources, Patrick searched for another way to understand human nutrition that was logical, consistent, and effective. His books on food and nutrition reflect this 'cleaner,' more intuitive and useful understanding of food and how it impacts our health.

Patrick hopes that his books will save his audience time and aggravation by finally offering practical ways to achieve their nutrition and fitness goals.

Made in the USA
Lexington, KY
23 November 2013